Exploring the relationship between inner city environments and Post-Traumatic Stress Disorder (PTSD) unveils a complex interplay of socio-economic factors, environmental stressors, and psychological mechanisms.

While traditionally associated with combat veterans or survivors of catastrophic events, PTSD can manifest in individuals living in urban settings due to chronic exposure to violence, poverty, discrimination, and other adversities endemic to these environments.

This book delves into the multifaceted nature of inner city PTSD, examining its root causes, symptomatology, and potential interventions.

The Urban Landscape: A Breeding Ground for Trauma

Inner city environments are often characterized by high levels of crime, gang activity, substance abuse, and socioeconomic disparities. The prevalence of these stressors creates an atmosphere ripe for the development of trauma-related disorders. Residents of such areas frequently experience or witness violence, including shootings, assaults, and domestic abuse, which can lead to a heightened sense of threat and vulnerability.

Additionally, systemic issues such as inadequate access to healthcare, education, and employment further compound the stressors faced by individuals living in inner cities.

The Impact of Chronic Stress

Exposure to chronic stressors in urban environments can dysregulate the body's stress response systems, leading to a plethora of physical and psychological health problems.

The hypothalamic-pituitary-adrenal (HPA) axis, responsible for regulating stress hormones like cortisol, may become overactive in response to prolonged stress, contributing to symptoms of anxiety, depression, and hypervigilance—all common features of PTSD.

Moreover, chronic stress can compromise immune function, exacerbating vulnerability to illness and disease.

Neighborhood Violence and PTSD

 One of the most significant contributors to PTSD in inner city environments is exposure to violence.

 Research indicates that individuals residing in violent neighborhoods are at a heightened risk of developing PTSD symptoms akin to those observed in combat veterans.

Witnessing or experiencing violence can evoke feelings of terror, helplessness, and horror—core features of traumatic events as defined by the Diagnostic and Statistical Manual of Mental Disorders (DSM-5).

Moreover, repeated exposure to trauma can lead to desensitization, wherein individuals become numb to the effects of violence, further complicating their psychological well-being.

Complex Trauma and Interpersonal Relationships

In addition to community-level stressors, individuals living in inner cities may grapple with interpersonal traumas such as childhood abuse, neglect, or intimate partner violence.

These experiences, often rooted in systemic inequities and social marginalization, can profoundly impact one's sense of self-worth, safety, and trust in others.

Complex trauma, characterized by multiple and prolonged traumatic experiences, can manifest in a range of PTSD symptoms, including flashbacks, nightmares, emotional dysregulation, and dissociation.

Coping Mechanisms and Maladaptive Behaviors

To cope with the chronic stressors inherent in inner city life, individuals may resort to maladaptive coping strategies such as substance abuse, aggression, or avoidance.

While these behaviors may provide temporary relief from distress, they ultimately perpetuate the cycle of trauma by exacerbating social and psychological problems.

Substance abuse, for instance, not only serves as a form of self-medication but also increases the likelihood of exposure to further traumatic events, such as drug-related violence or overdose.

Barriers to Treatment and Healing

Despite the prevalence of PTSD in inner city populations, access to mental health services remains woefully inadequate.

Stigmatization of mental illness, lack of culturally competent care, and financial constraints often deter individuals from seeking help.

Moreover, systemic barriers such as under-resourced community mental health centers and limited insurance coverage further exacerbate disparities in access to care.

Consequently, many individuals suffering from inner city PTSD go undiagnosed and untreated, perpetuating cycles of trauma within their communities.

Interventions and Hope for Recovery

Addressing inner city PTSD necessitates a multi-faceted approach that acknowledges the intersecting factors contributing to trauma within these environments.

Community-based interventions that promote resilience, social support, and empowerment have shown promise in mitigating the impact of trauma in urban settings.

Trauma-informed care, which emphasizes safety, trustworthiness, choice, collaboration, and empowerment, can help create healing spaces for individuals affected by PTSD.

Additionally, efforts to address systemic inequalities, improve access to education and employment opportunities, and reduce neighborhood violence are crucial for preventing trauma and fostering community well-being.

In conclusion, inner city environments can indeed give rise to a form of PTSD characterized by chronic exposure to violence, poverty, and social marginalization.

Understanding the complex interplay of socio-economic factors, environmental stressors, and psychological mechanisms underlying inner city PTSD is paramount for developing effective interventions and fostering healing within these communities.

By addressing root causes and promoting resilience, we can work towards creating safer, more supportive environments where individuals can thrive despite the adversities they face.

I wrote this using Artificial Intelligence.

I did not write this to create excuses for urban issues but to spot causes that can be acknowledged and fixed if not at least coped with in a healthy way.

Hopefully this helps you identify the need to seek help if you feel you have been affected by Urban PTSD.

Please use the next few pages
for your notes and debates.

www.ingramcontent.com/pod-product-compliance
Lightning Source LLC
Chambersburg PA
CBHW061322250726
48653CB00002B/1000